Bread Machine Recipes

A Practical Approach To Delicious Foolproof Bread Machine Recipes For Weight Loss, Fat Burning, And Healthy Living

Giulia Baker

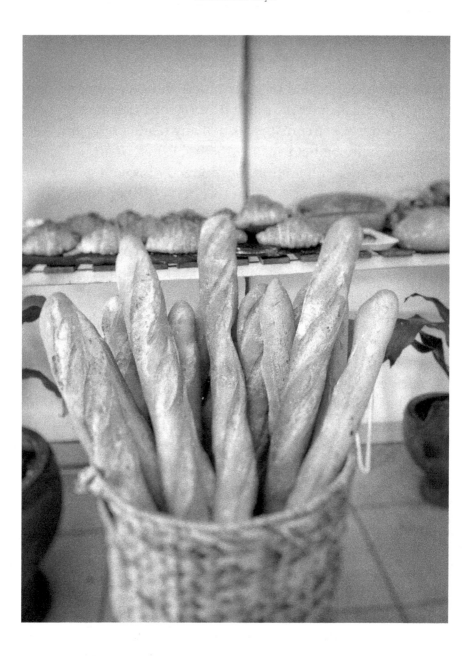

Table of Contents

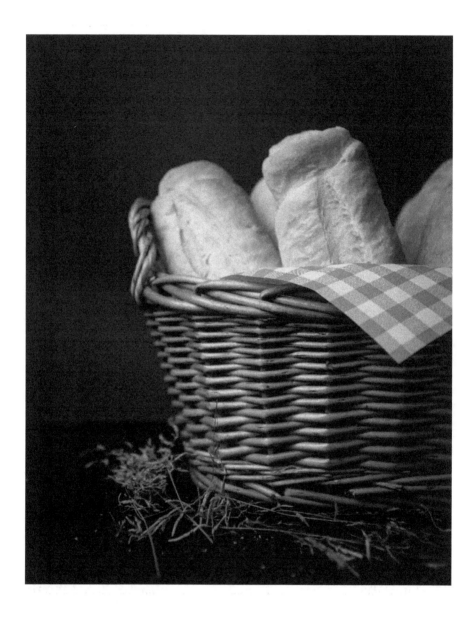

Introduction

Since then we all love bread, before we discover fire, it has been on the menu and we enjoy it so much. But as time goes by, we replace fire and primitive cooking methods with bread machine, from traditional baking to modern baking.

Modern baking using bread machines are more conventional to people who are always on the go. They are also invented to make baking more a lot easier. Considering what type of bread machine to consider will be depending on the volume you always you make. Time to time there will always be new technologies on bread machine but they all give you positive result- yummy bread.

Healthy and tasty bread surely is made from the best quality ingredients. Not only the freshest things that you can put in the mixing bowl, but the right cooking process also determine the delicacy and the safety of the bread.

Basically, bread is made from flour, water, yeast, and salt. After measuring the ingredients according to the recipe, the second step of making bread is mixing the ingredients. This step can be done using a mixer or manually kneading by hands. No matter what tool do you use, the dough should reach the right consistency. After the dough reaches the right consistency, the dough will be left to sit for a period of time to allow the fermentation process. Once it rises to double its size, it should be punched to expel the air inside the dough. Next, it is time to divide and fill the dough according to the baker's desire. After that, the filled dough should be sat for the final fermentation and later, bake the bread.

Well, making bread seems to be a long way to go. There are many steps to take in order to get soft and yummy bread. The right consistency of the dough is the first main key to generate perfect bread. However, this step is slightly tricky, and often makes people fail in making bread. One way to check the right consistency is by stretching a little bit of the dough. If the dough is stretched, it will become wide, transparent, and will not rip. If the dough doesn't reach the proper consistency, hard bread will certainly be resulted.

Luckily, a bread machine comes to be the best partner for every amateur baker who wants to bake bread from home. As a true assistant, the bread machine not only shortens the steps of making bread, but it also makes the process a lot easier. You just need to put the ingredients inside the baking tin, cover the bread machine, and hit the buttons. The bread machine ensures you to get the perfect bread that is usually found in famous bakeries. The great thing about this appliance is that the bread machine does all the bread making process for you, unattended. While you are waiting for the bread machine do its job, you still can do all your daily activities or enjoy your favorite movie.

Making bread seemed to be so impossible that most people never dreamed of doing so. However, a bread machine changes it all. Now, millions of people turn their lovely kitchen to bakeries. Everyone can enjoy the freshest, healthiest, and tastiest bread from their own warm kitchen without spending too much money for it.

The most beneficial of having a bread machine is having fresh bread at the tip of your finger. You just need to prepare the necessary ingredients ahead of time, and let the machine do the work.

Secondly, you can control the ingredients, add delicious ingredients that suits to your palate.

Bread machines make more than bread. Bread machine is not just for making breads; you can use it to make jam, pasta and dough for your homemade pizza.

Superior taste and quality of bread, they are easy to operate. So you don't have to worry whether you are a good baker or not. Bread machines are programmed to make perfect heavenly breads. Same process in traditional making of bread you must also consider following instructions and considering that you are using a machine the right settings in cooking bread. Baking using bread machine will also bring out one's creativity.

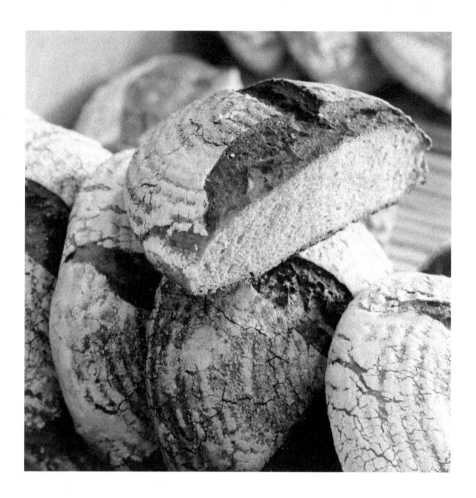

Basic Breads

1. Basic White Bread

Preparation Time: 1 hour 15 minutes

Cooking Time: 50 minutes (20+30 minutes)

Servings: 1 loaf

Ingredients:

½ to 5/8 cup Water 5/8 cup Milk

1 ½ tablespoon butter or margarine

3 tablespoon Sugar

1 ½ teaspoon Salt

3 cups Bread Flour

1 ½ teaspoon Active dry Yeast

Directions:

Put all ingredients in the bread pan, using minimal measure of liquid listed in the recipe.

Select medium Crust setting and press Start.

Observe the dough as it kneads. Following 5 to 10 minutes, in the event that it seems dry and firm, or if your machine seems as though it's straining to knead, add more liquid 1 tablespoon at a time until dough forms well.

Once the baking cycle ends, remove bread from pan, and allow to cool before slicing.

Calories: 64 Cal

Fat: 1 g

Carbohydrates: 12 g

Protein: 2 g

2. Gluten Free Bread

Preparation Time: 4 hour 50 minutes

Cooking Time: 50 minutes (20+30 minutes)

Servings: 1 loaf

Ingredients:

2 cups rice flour Potato starch

1/2 cup Tapioca flour

1/2 cup Xanthan gum

2 1/2 teaspoons 2/3 cup powdered milk or 1/2 non diary substitute

1 1/2 teaspoons Salt

1 1/2 teaspoons egg substitute (optional)

3 tablespoons Sugar

1 2/3 cups lukewarm water

1 1/2 tablespoons Dry yeast, granules

4 tablespoons Butter, melted or margarine

1 teaspoon Vinegar

3 eggs, room temperature

Directions:

Add yeast to the bread pan.

Add all the flours, xanthan/ gum, milk powder, salt, and sugar.

Beat the eggs, and mix with water, butter, and vinegar.

Choose white bread setting at medium or use 3-4 hour setting.

Nutrition:

Calories: 126 Cal

Fat   : 2 g

Carbohydrates: 29 g

Protein : 3 g

3. All-Purpose White Bread

Preparation Time: 2 hours 10 minutes

Cooking Time: 40 minutes

Servings: 1 loaf

Ingredients:

¾ cup water at 80 degrees F

1 tablespoon melted butter, cooled

1 tablespoon sugar

¾ teaspoon salt 2 tablespoons skim milk powder

2 cups white bread flour

¾ teaspoon instant yeast

Directions:

Add all of the ingredients to your bread machine, carefully following the instructions of the manufacturer.

Set the program of your bread machine to Basic/White Bread and set

crust type to Medium.

Press START.

Wait until the cycle completes.

Once the loaf is ready, take the bucket out and let the loaf cool for 5

minutes.

Gently shake the bucket to remove the loaf.

Put to a cooling rack, slice, and serve.

Nutrition:

Calories: 140 Cal

Fat: 2 g

Carbohydrates: 27 g

Protein: 44 g

Fiber: 2 g

4. Mustard-Flavored General Bread

Preparation Time: 2 hours 10 minutes

Cooking Time: 40 minutes

Servings: 2 loaves

Ingredients:

1¼ cups milk 3 tablespoons sunflower milk

3 tablespoons sour cream

2 tablespoons dry mustard

1 whole egg, beaten

½ sachet sugar vanilla

4 cups flour 1 teaspoon dry yeast

2 tablespoons sugar 2 teaspoon salt

Directions:

Take out the bread maker's bucket and pour in milk and sunflower oil;

stir and then add sour cream and beaten egg.

Add flour, salt, sugar, mustard powder, vanilla sugar, and mix well.

Make a small groove in the flour and sprinkle the yeast.

Transfer the bucket to your bread maker and cover.

Set the program of your bread machine to Basic/White Bread and set crust type to Medium.

Press START.

Wait until the cycle completes.

Once the loaf is ready, take the bucket out and let the loaf cool for 5 minutes.

Gently shake the bucket to remove the loaf.

Transfer to a cooling rack, slice, and serve.

Nutrition:

Calories: 340 Cal Fat: 10 g Carbohydrates:54 g

Protein: 10 g Fiber: 1 g

Fiber: 1 g

5. Country White Bread

Preparation Time: 3 hours

Cooking Time: 45 minutes

Servings: 2 loaves

Ingredients:

2 teaspoon active dry yeast

1 1/2 tablespoon sugar

4 cups bread flour

1 1/2 teaspoon salt

1 large egg 1 1/2 tablespoon butter

1 cup warm milk, with a temperature of 110 to 115 degrees F (43 to 46

degrees C)

Directions:

Put all the liquid ingredients in the pan. Add all the dry ingredients,

except the yeast. Use your hand to form a hole in the middle of the dry ingredients. Put the yeast in the hole.

Secure the pan in the chamber and close the lid. Choose the basic setting

and your preferred crust color. Press start.

Once done, transfer the baked bread to a wire rack. Slice once cooled.

Nutrition:

Calories: 105 calories;

Total Carbohydrate: 0 g

Total Fat: 0 g

Protein: 0 g

6. Oatmeal Bread

Preparation Time: 3 hours

Cooking Time: 45 minutes

Servings: 2 loaves

Ingredients:

3 teaspoon bread machine yeast

4 teaspoon vital wheat gluten

4 cups bread flour

1 teaspoon salt

1 cup instant or regular oatmeal

2 tablespoon maple syrup

2 tablespoon unsalted butter, cubed

1/3 cup water, with a temperature of 80 to 90 degrees F (26 to 32 degrees C)

1 1/2 cups buttermilk, with a temperature of 80 to 90 degrees F (26 to 32 degrees C)

Directions:

Put the ingredients in the pan in this order: buttermilk, water, butter, maple syrup, oatmeal, salt, flour, gluten, and yeast.

Secure the pan in the machine, close the lid and turn it on.

Choose the basic setting and your preferred crust color and press start.

Transfer the baked bread to a wire rack and allow to cool before slicing.

Nutrition:

Calories: 269 calories;

Total Carbohydrate: 49 g

Total Fat: 4 g

Protein: 8 g

Spice and Herb Breads

7. Herb Bread

Preparation Time: 1 hour 20 minutes

Cooking Time: 50 minutes (20+30 minutes)

Servings: 1 loaf

Ingredients:

3/4 to 7/8 cup milk

1 tablespoon Sugar

1 teaspoon Salt

2 tablespoon Butter or margarine

1/3 cup chopped onion

2 cups bread flour

1/2 teaspoon Dried dill

1/2 teaspoon Dried basil

1/2 teaspoon Dried rosemary

11/2 teaspoon Active dry yeast

Directions:

Place all the Ingredients in the bread pan. Select medium crus then the

rapid bake cycle. Press start.

After 5-10 minutes, observe the dough as it kneads, if you hear straining

sounds in your machine or if the dough appears stiff and dry, add 1

tablespoon Liquid at a time until the dough becomes smooth, pliable,

soft, and slightly tacky to the touch.

Remove the bread from the pan after baking. Place on rack and allow

to cool for 1 hour before slicing.

Nutrition:

Calories: 65 Cal Fat: 0 g Carbohydrates:13 g

Protein : 2 g

8. Awesome Rosemary Bread

Preparation Time: 2 hours 10 minutes

Cooking Time: 50 minutes

Servings: 1 loaf

Ingredients:

¾ cup + 1 tablespoon water at 80 degrees F

1⅔ tablespoons melted butter, cooled

2 teaspoons sugar

1 teaspoon salt 1 tablespoon fresh rosemary, chopped

2 cups white bread flour

1⅓ teaspoons instant yeast

Directions:

Add all of the ingredients to your bread machine, carefully following the

instructions of the manufacturer.

Set the program of your bread machine to Basic/White Bread and set

crust type to Medium.

Press START.

Wait until the cycle completes.

Once the loaf is ready, take the bucket out and let the loaf cool for 5

minutes.

Gently shake the bucket to remove the loaf.

Transfer to a cooling rack, slice, and serve.

Nutrition:

Calories: 142 Cal

Fat: 3 g

Carbohydrates: 25 g

Protein: 4 g

Fiber: 1 g

9. Original Italian Herb Bread

Preparation Time: 2 hours 40 minutes

Cooking Time: 50 minutes

Servings: 2 loaves

Ingredients:

1 cup water at 80 degrees F

½ cup olive brine 1½ tablespoons butter

3 tablespoons sugar   teaspoons salt

5⅓ cups flour

2 teaspoons bread machine yeast

20 olives, black/green 1½ teaspoons Italian herbs

Directions:

Cut olives into slices.

Add all of the ingredients to your bread machine (except olives), carefully following the instructions of the manufacturer.

Set the program of your bread machine to French bread and set crust type to Medium.

Press START.

Once the maker beeps, add olives.

Wait until the cycle completes.

Once the loaf is ready, take the bucket out and let the loaf cool for 5 minutes.

Gently shake the bucket to remove the loaf.

Transfer to a cooling rack, slice, and serve.

Nutrition:

Calories: 386 Cal

Fat: 7 g Carbohydrates:71 g

Protein: 10 g

Fiber: 1 g

10.Lovely Aromatic Lavender Bread

Preparation Time: 2 hours 10 minutes

Cooking Time: 50 minutes

Servings: 1 loaf

Ingredients:

¾ cup milk at 80 degrees F

1 tablespoon melted butter, cooled

1 tablespoon sugar

¾ teaspoon salt

1 teaspoon fresh lavender flower, chopped

¼ teaspoon lemon zest

¼ teaspoon fresh thyme, chopped

2 cups white bread flour

¾ teaspoon instant yeast

Directions:

Add all of the ingredients to your bread machine

Set the program of your bread machine to Basic/White Bread and set crust type to Medium.

Press START.

Wait until the cycle completes.

Once the loaf is ready, take the bucket out and let the loaf cool for 5 minutes.

Gently shake the bucket to remove the loaf.

Transfer to a cooling rack, slice, and serve.

Nutrition:

Calories: 144 Cal

Fat: 2 g

Carbohydrates: 27 g

Protein: 4 g

Fiber: 1 g

11. Oregano Mozza-Cheese Bread

Preparation Time: 2 hours 50 minutes

Cooking Time: 50 minutes

Servings: 2 loaves

Ingredients:

1 cup (milk + egg) mixture

½ cup mozzarella cheese

2¼ cups flour

¾ cup whole grain flour

2 tablespoons sugar

1 teaspoon salt 2 teaspoons oregano

1½ teaspoons dry yeast

Directions:

Add all of the ingredients to your bread machine

Set the program of your bread machine to Basic/White Bread and set crust type to Dark.

Press START.

Wait until the cycle completes.

Once the loaf is ready, take the bucket out and let the loaf cool for 5 minutes.

Gently shake the bucket to remove the loaf.

Transfer to a cooling rack, slice, and serve.

Nutrition:

Calories: 209 Cal

Fat: 2.1 g

Carbohydrates: 40 g

Protein: 7.7 g

Fiber: 1 g

12.Garlic Bread

Preparation Time: 2 hours 30 minutes

Cooking Time: 40 minutes

Servings: 1 loaf

Ingredients:

1 3/8 cups water

3 tablespoons olive oil

1 teaspoon minced garlic

4 cups bread flour

3 tablespoons white sugar

2 teaspoons salt

1/4 cup grated Parmesan cheese

1 teaspoon dried basil

1 teaspoon garlic powder

3 tablespoons chopped fresh chives

1 teaspoon coarsely ground black pepper

2 1/2 teaspoons bread machine yeast

Directions:

Follow the order of putting the ingredients into the pan of the bread

machine recommended by the manufacturer.

Choose the Basic or the White Bread cycle on the machine and press

the Start button.

Nutrition:

Calories: 175 calories;

Total Carbohydrate: 29.7 g

Cholesterol: 1 mg

Total Fat: 3.7 g

Protein: 5.2 g

Sodium: 332 mg

13.Rosemary Bread

Preparation Time: 2 hours 40 minutes

Cooking Time: 25- 30 minutes

Servings: 1 loaf

Ingredients:

1 cup water

3 tablespoons olive oil

1 1/2 teaspoons white sugar

1 1/2 teaspoons salt

1/4 teaspoon Italian seasoning

1/4 teaspoon ground black pepper

1 tablespoon dried rosemary

2 1/2 cups bread flour

1 1/2 teaspoons active dry yeast

Directions:

Into the bread machine pan, put the ingredients following the order recommended by manufacturer. Use the white bread cycle and then push the Start button.

Nutrition:

Calories: 137 calories;

Total Carbohydrate: 21.6 g

Cholesterol: 0 mg

Total Fat: 3.9 g

Protein: 3.6 g

Sodium: 292 mg

Grain, Seed and Nut Bread

14.Cracked Wheat Bread

Preparation Time: 3 hours 5 minutes

Cooking Time: 15 minutes

Servings: 12

Ingredients:

1 1/4 cups water

2 tablespoons margarine, softened

2 tablespoons dry milk powder

2 tablespoons brown sugar

1 1/4 teaspoons salt

3 cups bread flour

1/3 cup whole wheat flour

1/4 cup cracked wheat

1 1/4 teaspoons active dry yeast

Directions:

In bread machine pan, measure all of the ingredients in the order the manufacturer suggested. Choose regular/light cycle; then start.

Nutrition:

Calories: 50 calories;

Total Carbohydrate: 7.3 g

Cholesterol: < 1 mg

Total Fat: 1.9 g

Protein: 1.4 g

Sodium: 271 mg

Sodium: 189 mg

15.Flax and Sunflower Seed Bread

Preparation Time: 3 hours

Cooking Time: 15 minutes

Servings: 15

Ingredients:

1 1/3 cups water

2 tablespoons butter, softened

3 tablespoons honey

1 1/2 cups bread flour

1 1/3 cups whole wheat bread flour

1 teaspoon salt

1 teaspoon active dry yeast

1/2 cup flax seeds

1/2 cup sunflower seeds

Directions:

With suggested order by manufacturer, add the all ingredients, (apart from sunflower seeds) in pan of bread machine. Select basic white cycle; press start. Just in the knead cycle that your machine signals alert sounds, add the sunflower seeds.

Nutrition:

Calories: 140 calories;

Total Carbohydrate: 22.7 g

Cholesterol: 4 mg

Total Fat: 4.2 g

Protein: 4.2 g

Sodium: 169 mg

16.High Flavor Bran Bread

Preparation Time: 3 hours

Cooking Time: 15 minutes

Servings: 15

Ingredients:

1 1/2 cups warm water (110 degrees F/45 degrees C)

2 tablespoons dry milk powder

2 tablespoons vegetable oil

2 tablespoons molasses

2 tablespoons honey

1 1/2 teaspoons salt

2 1/4 cups whole wheat flour

1 1/4 cups bread flour

1 cup whole bran cereal

2 teaspoons active dry yeast

Directions:

In the pan of your bread machine, add the ingredients in the directed by the machine's maker. Set the machine to either the whole grain or whole wheat setting.

Nutrition:

Calories: 146 calories;

Total Carbohydrate: 27.9 g

Cholesterol: < 1 mg

Total Fat: 2.4 g

Protein: 4.6 g

Sodium: 254 mg

17.Honey and Flaxseed Bread

Preparation Time: 3 hours

Cooking Time: 15 minutes

Servings: 12

Ingredients:

1 1/8 cups water

1 1/2 tablespoons flaxseed oil

3 tablespoons honey

1/2 tablespoon liquid lecithin

3 cups whole wheat flour

1/2 cup flax seed

2 tablespoons bread flour

3 tablespoons whey powder

1 1/2 teaspoons sea salt

2 teaspoons active dry yeast

Directions:

In the bread machine pan, put in all of the ingredients following the order recommended by the manufacturer.

Choose the Wheat cycle on the machine and press the Start button to run the machine.

Nutrition:

Calories: 174 calories;

Total Carbohydrate: 30.8 g

Cholesterol: < 1 mg

Total Fat: 4.9 g

Protein: 7.1 g

Sodium: 242 mg

18.Honey Whole Wheat Bread

Preparation Time: 3 hours 5 minutes

Cooking Time: 15 minutes

Servings: 10

Ingredients:

1 1/8 cups warm water (110 degrees F/45 degrees C)

3 tablespoons honey 1/3 teaspoon salt

1 1/2 cups whole wheat flour

1 1/2 cups bread flour

2 tablespoons vegetable oil

1 1/2 teaspoons active dry yeast

Directions:

Put the ingredients into the bread machine following the order recommended by the manufacturer. Choose the Wheat Bread cycle and the setting for Light Color on the machine.

Nutrition:

Calories: 180 calories;

Total Carbohydrate: 33.4 g

Cholesterol: 0 mg

Total Fat: 3.5 g

Protein: 5.2 g

Sodium: 79 mg

19.Maple Whole Wheat Bread

Preparation Time: 3 hours 5 minutes

Cooking Time: 15 minutes

Servings: 10

Ingredients:

2 1/2 cups whole wheat flour

1/2 cup bread flour

1/3 teaspoon salt 1 1/4 cups water

4 tablespoons maple syrup

2 tablespoons olive oil

1 1/2 teaspoons active dry yeast

Directions:

Put the ingredients into the bread machine pan following the order suggested by the manufacturer. Choose the Wheat Bread cycle on the machine and press the Start button.

Nutrition:

Calories: 144 calories;

Total Carbohydrate: 26.9 g

Cholesterol: 0 mg

Total Fat: 2.8 g

Protein: 4.3 g

Sodium: 67 mg

20. Oat and Honey Bread

Preparation Time: 3 hours 5 minutes

Cooking Time: 15 minutes

Servings: 10

Ingredients:

1 cup buttermilk

1 egg

1/4 cup warm water (110 degrees F/45 degrees C)

2 tablespoons honey

1 1/2 cups whole wheat flour

1 1/2 cups all-purpose flour

1/2 cup quick cooking oats

2 tablespoons vegetable oil

1 1/2 teaspoons salt

1 1/2 teaspoons active dry yeast

Directions:

Check all ingredients and place them into the bread machine according

to the manufacturer's suggestion.

Select Light Crust or Whole Wheat. Press Start.

Nutrition:

Calories: 200 calories;

Total Carbohydrate: 35 g

Cholesterol: 20 mg

Total Fat: 4.3 g

Protein: 6.6 g

Sodium: 384 mg

Cheese Bread

21. Onion, Garlic, Cheese Bread

Preparation Time: 50 minutes

Cooking Time: 40 minutes

Servings: 1 loaf

Ingredients:

3 tablespoon Dried minced onion

3 cups bread flour

2 teaspoon Garlic powder

2 teaspoon Active dry yeast

2 tablespoon White sugar

2 tablespoon Margarine

2 tablespoon Dry milk powder

1 cup shredded sharp cheddar cheese

1 1/8 cups warm water

1 1/2 teaspoon Salt

Directions:

In the order suggested by the manufacturer, put the flour, water, powdered milk, margarine or butter, salt, and yeast in the bread pan.

Press the basic cycle with light crust. When the sound alerts or as directed by the manufacturer, add 2 teaspoon Of the onion flakes, the garlic powder, and all of the shredded cheese.

After the last kneed, sprinkle the remaining onion flakes over the dough.

Nutrition:

Calories: 204 calories;

Total Carbohydrate: 29 g

Total Fat: 6 g

Protein: 8 g

22. Cream Cheese Bread

Preparation Time: 60 minutes

Cooking Time: 35 minutes

Servings: 1 loaf

Ingredients:

1/2 cup Water

1/2 cup Cream cheese, softened

2 tablespoons Melted butter

1 Beaten egg 4 tablespoons Sugar

1 teaspoon Salt

3 cups Bread flour

1 1/2 teaspoons Active dry yeast

Directions:

Place the ingredients in the pan in the order as suggested by your bread

machine

Manufacturer.

Process on dough cycle.

Remove from machine, form into a loaf and place in greased 9x5 loaf pan.

Cover and let rise until doubled.

Bake in a 350° oven for approximately 35 minutes.

Nutrition:

Calories: 150 calories;

Total Carbohydrate: 24 g

Total Fat: 5 g

Protein: 3 g

23. Mozzarella Cheese and Salami Loaf

Preparation Time: 2 hours 50 minutes

Cooking Time: 45 minutes

Servings: 1 loaf

Ingredients:

¾ cup water, at 80 degrees F

1/3 cup mozzarella cheese, shredded

4 teaspoons sugar

2/3 teaspoon salt

2/3 teaspoon dried basil

Pinch of garlic powder

2 cups + 2 tablespoons white bread flour

1 teaspoon instant yeast ½ cup hot salami, finely diced

Directions:

Add the listed ingredients to your bread machine (except salami), following the manufactures instructions.

Set the bread machine's program to Basic/White Bread and the crust type to Light. Press Start.

Let the bread machine work and wait until it beeps, this your indication to add the remaining ingredients. At this point add the salami.

Wait until the remaining bake cycle completes.

Once the loaf is done, take the bucket out from the bread machine and let it rest for 5 minutes.

Gently shake the bucket and remove the loaf, transfer the loaf to a cooling rack and slice.

Serve and enjoy!

Nutrition:

Calories: 164 calories; Total Carbohydrate: 28 g

Total Fat: 3 g Protein: 6 g

Sugar: 2 g

24. Olive and Cheddar Loaf

Preparation Time: 2 hours 50 minutes

Cooking Time: 45 minutes

Servings: 1 loaf

Ingredients:

1 cup water, room temperature

4 teaspoons sugar

¾ teaspoon salt

1 and 1/ cups sharp cheddar cheese, shredded

3 cups bread flour

2 teaspoons active dry yeast

¾ cup pimiento olives, drained and sliced

Directions:

Add the listed ingredients to your bread machine (except salami), following the manufactures instructions.

Set the bread machine's program to Basic/White Bread and the crust type to Light. Press Start.

Let the bread machine work and wait until it beeps, this your indication to add the remaining ingredients. At this point add the salami.

Wait until the remaining bake cycle completes.

Once the loaf is done, take the bucket out from the bread machine and let it rest for 5 minutes.

Gently shake the bucket and remove the loaf, transfer the loaf to a cooling rack and slice.

Serve and enjoy!

Nutrition:

Calories: 124 calories;

Total Carbohydrate: 19 g

Total Fat: 4 g Protein: 5 g

Sugar: 5 g

25. Cottage Cheese Bread

Preparation Time: 2 hours 50 minutes

Cooking Time: 45 minutes

Servings: 1 loaf

Ingredients:

1/2 cup water

1 cup cottage cheese

2 tablespoons margarine

1 egg 1 tablespoon white sugar

1/4 teaspoon baking soda

1 teaspoon salt 3 cups bread flour

2 1/2 teaspoons active dry yeast

Directions:

Into the bread machine, place the ingredients according to the order

recommended by manufacturer and then push the start button. In case the dough looks too sticky, feel free to use up to half cup more bread flour.

Nutrition:

Calories: 171 calories;

Total Carbohydrate: 26.8 g

Cholesterol: 18 mg

Total Fat: 3.6 g

Protein: 7.3 g

Sodium: 324 mg

26. Green Cheese Bread

Preparation Time: 3 hours

Cooking Time: 15 minutes

Servings: 8

Ingredients:

¾ cup lukewarm water 1 Tablespoon sugar

1 teaspoon kosher salt 2 Tablespoon green cheese

1 cup wheat bread machine flour

9/10 cup whole-grain flour, finely ground

1 teaspoon bread machine yeast

1 teaspoon ground paprika

Directions:

Place all the dry and liquid ingredients, except paprika, in the pan and

follow the instructions for your bread machine.

Pay particular attention to measuring the ingredients. Use a measuring cup, measuring spoon, and kitchen scales to do so.

Dissolve yeast in warm milk in a saucepan and add in the last turn.

Add paprika after the beep or place it in the dispenser of the bread machine. Set the baking program to BASIC and the crust type to DARK. If the dough is too dense or too wet, adjust the amount of flour and liquid in the recipe.

When the program has ended, take the pan out of the bread machine and let cool for 5 minutes.

Shake the loaf out of the pan. If necessary, use a spatula.

Wrap the bread with a kitchen towel and set it aside for an hour. Otherwise, you can cool it on a wire rack.

Nutrition:

Calories: 118 calories; Total Carbohydrate: 23.6 g Cholesterol: 2 g

Total Fat: 1 g Protein: 4.1 g Sodium: 304 mg Sugar: 1.6 g

Fiber: 1 g

Fruit Breads

27. Banana Bread

Preparation Time: 1 hour 40 minutes

Cooking Time: 40- 45 minutes

Servings: 1 loaf

Ingredients:

1 teaspoon Baking powder

1/2 teaspoon Baking soda

2 bananas, peeled and halved lengthwise

2 cups all-purpose flour

2 eggs

3 tablespoon Vegetable oil

3/4 cup white sugar

Directions:

Put all the Ingredients in the bread pan. Select dough setting. Start and mix for about 3-5 minutes.

After 3-5 minutes, press stop. Do not continue to mix. Smooth out the top of the dough

Using the spatula and then select bake, start and bake for about 50 minutes. After 50 minutes, insert a toothpick into the top center to test doneness.

Test the loaf again. When the bread is completely baked, remove the pan from the machine and let the bread remain in the pan for10 minutes. Remove bread and cool in wire rack.

Nutrition:

Calories: 310 calories Total Carbohydrate: 40 g

Fat: 13 g Protein: 3 g

28. Blueberry Bread

Preparation Time: 3 hours 15 minutes

Cooking Time: 40- 45 minutes

Servings: 1 loaf

Ingredients:

1⅛ to 1¼ cups Water 6 ounces Cream cheese, softened

2 tablespoons Butter or margarine

¼ cup Sugar 2 teaspoons Salt

4½ cups Bread flour

1½ teaspoons Grated lemon peel

2 teaspoons Cardamom

2 tablespoons Nonfat dry milk

2½ teaspoons Red star brand active dry yeast

⅔ cup dried blueberries

Directions:

Place all Ingredients except dried blueberries in bread pan, using the least amount of liquid listed in the recipe. Select light crust setting and raisin/nut cycle. Press start.

Observe the dough as it kneads. After 5 to 10 minutes, if it appears dry and stiff or if your ma- chine sounds as if it's straining to knead it, add more liquid 1 tablespoon at a time until dough forms a smooth, soft, pliable ball that is slightly tacky to the touch.

At the beep, add the dried blueberries.

After the baking cycle ends, remove bread from pan, place on cake rack, and allow to cool 1 hour before slicing.

Nutrition:

Calories: 180 calories Total Carbohydrate: 250 g

Fat: 3 g Protein: 9 g

29. Orange and Walnut Bread

Preparation Time: 2 hours 50 minutes

Cooking Time: 45 minutes

Servings: 10- 15

Ingredients:

1 egg white

1 tablespoon water

½ cup warm whey

1 tablespoons yeast

4 tablespoons sugar

2 oranges, crushed

4 cups flour

1 teaspoon salt

1 and ½ tablespoon salt

3 teaspoons orange peel

1/3 teaspoon vanilla

3 tablespoons walnut and almonds, crushed

Crushed pepper, salt, cheese for garnish

Directions:

Add all of the ingredients to your Bread Machine (except egg white, 1 tablespoon water and crushed pepper/ cheese).

Set the program to "Dough" cycle and let the cycle run.

Remove the dough (using lightly floured hands) and carefully place it on a floured surface.

Cover with a light film/cling paper and let the dough rise for 10 minutes.

Divide the dough into thirds after it has risen

Place on a lightly flour surface, roll each portion into 14x10 inch sized rectangles

Use a sharp knife to cut carefully cut the dough into strips of ½ inch width

Pick 2-3 strips and twist them multiple times, making sure to press the ends together

Preheat your oven to 400 degrees F

Take a bowl and stir egg white, water and brush onto the breadsticks

Sprinkle salt, pepper/ cheese

Bake for 10-12 minutes until golden brown

Remove from baking sheet and transfer to cooling rack Serve and enjoy!

Nutrition:

Calories: 437 calories;

Total Carbohydrate: 82 g

Total Fat: 7 g

Protein: 12 g

Sugar: 34 g

Fiber: 1 g

30. Lemon and Poppy Buns

Preparation Time: 2 hours 50 minutes

Cooking Time: 45 minutes

Servings: 10- 20 buns

Ingredients:

Melted Butter for grease 1 and 1/3 cups hot water

3 tablespoons powdered milk 2 tablespoons Crisco shortening

1 and ½ teaspoon salt 1 tablespoon lemon juice

4 and ¼ cups bread flour ½ teaspoon nutmeg

2 teaspoons grated lemon rind

2 tablespoons poppy seeds

1 and ¼ teaspoons yeast

2 teaspoons wheat gluten

Directions:

Add all of the ingredients to your Bread Machine (except melted butter).

Set the program to "Dough" cycle and let the cycle run.

Remove the dough (using lightly floured hands) and carefully place it on a floured surface.

Cover with a light film/cling paper and let the dough rise for 10 minutes.

Take a large cookie sheet and grease with butter.

Cut the risen dough into 15-20 pieces and shape them into balls.

Place the balls onto the sheet (2 inches apart) and cover.

Place in a warm place and let them rise for 30-40 minutes until the dough doubles.

Preheat your oven to 375 degrees F, transfer the cookie sheet to your oven and bake for 12-15 minutes. Brush the top with a bit of butter, enjoy!

Nutrition:

Calories: 231 calories; Total Carbohydrate: 31 g Total Fat: 11 g

Protein: 4 g Sugar: 12 g Fiber: 1 g

31.Apple with Pumpkin Bread

Preparation Time: 2 hours 50 minutes

Cooking Time: 45 minutes **Servings:** 2 loaves

Ingredients:

1/3 cup dried apples, chopped

1 1/2 teaspoon bread machine yeast

4 cups bread flour 1/3 cup ground pecans

1/4 teaspoon ground nutmeg 1/4 teaspoon ground ginger

1/4 teaspoon allspice 1/2 teaspoon ground cinnamon

1 1/4 teaspoon salt 2 tablespoon unsalted butter, cubed

1/3 cup dry skim milk powder

1/4 cup honey

2 large eggs, at room temperature

2/3 cup pumpkin puree

2/3 cup water, with a temperature of 80 to 90 degrees F (26 to 32 degrees C)

Directions:

Put all ingredients, except the dried apples, in the bread pan in this order:

water, pumpkin puree, eggs, honey, skim milk, butter, salt, allspice,

cinnamon, pecans, nutmeg, ginger, flour, and yeast.

Secure the pan in the machine and lock the lid.

Place the dried apples in the fruit and nut dispenser.

Turn on the machine. Choose the sweet setting and your desired color

of the crust.

Carefully unmold the baked bread once done and allow to cool for 20

minutes before slicing.

Nutrition:

Calories: 228 calories; Total Carbohydrate: 30 g

Total Fat: 4 g Protein: 18 g

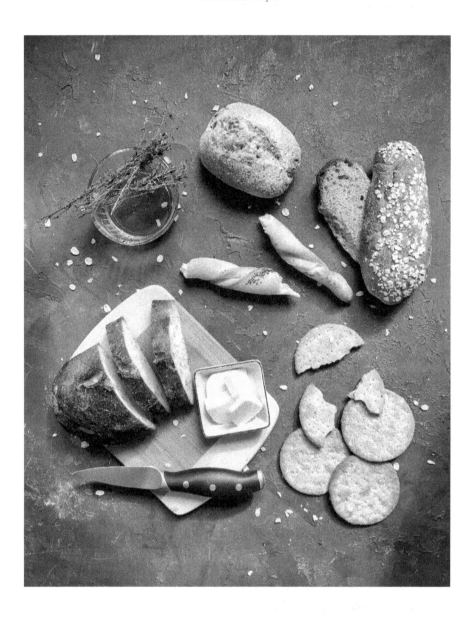

Vegetable Breads

32.   Healthy Celery Loaf

Preparation Time: 2 hours 40 minutes

Cooking Time: 50 minutes

Servings: 1 loaf

Ingredients:

1 can (10 ounces) cream of celery soup

3 tablespoons low-fat milk, heated

1 tablespoon vegetable oil

1¼ teaspoons celery salt

¾ cup celery, fresh/sliced thin

1 tablespoon celery leaves, fresh, chopped

1 whole egg

¼ teaspoon sugar

3 cups bread flour

¼ teaspoon ginger

½ cup quick-cooking oats

2 tablespoons gluten

2 teaspoons celery seeds

1 pack of active dry yeast

Directions:

Add all of the ingredients to your bread machine, carefully following the

instructions of the manufacturer

Set the program of your bread machine to Basic/White Bread and set

crust type to Medium

Press START

Wait until the cycle completes

Once the loaf is ready, take the bucket out and let the loaf cool for 5

minutes

Gently shake the bucket to remove the loaf

Transfer to a cooling rack, slice and serve

Enjoy!

Nutrition:

Calories: 73 Cal

Fat   : 4 g

Carbohydrates: 8 g

Protein : 3 g

Fiber: 1 g

33.   Broccoli and Cauliflower Bread

Preparation Time: 2 hours 20 minutes

Cooking Time: 50 minutes

Servings: 1 loaf

Ingredients:

¼ cup water

4 tablespoons olive oil

1 egg white

1 teaspoon lemon juice

2/3 cup grated cheddar cheese

3 tablespoons green onion

½ cup broccoli, chopped

½ cup cauliflower, chopped

½ teaspoon lemon pepper seasoning

2 cups bread flour

1 teaspoon bread machine yeast

Directions:

Add all of the ingredients to your bread machine, carefully following the

instructions of the manufacturer

Set the program of your bread machine to Basic/White Bread and set

crust type to Medium

Press START

Wait until the cycle completes

Once the loaf is ready, take the bucket out and let the loaf cool for 5

minutes

Gently shake the bucket to remove the loaf

Transfer to a cooling rack, slice and serve

Nutrition:

Calories: 156 Cal Fat: 8 g Carbohydrates:17 g

Protein: 5 g Fiber: 2 g

34. Zucchini Herbed Bread

Preparation Time: 2 hours 20 minutes

Cooking Time: 50 minutes

Servings: 1 loaf

Ingredients:

½ cup water

2 teaspoon honey

1 tablespoons oil

¾ cup zucchini, grated

¾ cup whole wheat flour

2 cups bread flour

1 tablespoon fresh basil, chopped

2 teaspoon sesame seeds

1 teaspoon salt

1½ teaspoon active dry yeast

Directions:

Add all of the ingredients to your bread machine, carefully following the instructions of the manufacturer

Set the program of your bread machine to Basic/White Bread and set crust type to Medium

Press START

Wait until the cycle completes

Once the loaf is ready, take the bucket out and let the loaf cool for 5 minutes

Gently shake the bucket to remove the loaf

Transfer to a cooling rack, slice and serve

Enjoy!

Nutrition:

Calories: 153 Cal Fat: 1 g Carbohydrates:28 g

Protein: 5 g Fiber: g

35. Potato Bread

Preparation Time: 3 hours

Cooking Time: 45 minutes

Servings: 2 loaves

Ingredients:

1 3/4 teaspoon active dry yeast

2 tablespoon dry milk

1/4 cup instant potato flakes

2 tablespoon sugar

4 cups bread flour 1 1/4 teaspoon salt

2 tablespoon butter 1 3/8 cups water

Directions:

Put all the liquid ingredients in the pan. Add all the dry ingredients, except the yeast. Form a shallow hole in the middle of the dry ingredients and place the yeast.

Secure the pan in the machine and close the lid. Choose the basic setting

and your desired color of the crust. Press start.

Allow the bread to cool before slicing.

Nutrition:

Calories: 35calories;

Total Carbohydrate: 19 g

Total Fat: 0 g

Protein: 4 g

36.   Golden Potato Bread

Preparation Time: 2 hours 50 minutes

Cooking Time: 45 minutes **Servings:** 2 loaves

Ingredients:

2 teaspoon bread machine yeast

3 cups bread flour 1 1/2 teaspoon salt

2 tablespoon potato starch

1 tablespoon dried chives

3 tablespoon dry skim milk powder

1 teaspoon sugar 2 tablespoon unsalted butter, cubed

3/4 cup mashed potatoes 1 large egg, at room temperature

3/4 cup potato cooking water, with a temperature of 80 to 90 degrees

F (26 to 32 degrees C)

Directions:

Prepare the mashed potatoes. Peel the potatoes and put them in a saucepan. Pour enough cold water to cover them. Turn the heat to high and bring to a boil. Turn the heat to low and continue cooking the potatoes until tender. Transfer the cooked potatoes to a bowl and mash. Cover the bowl until the potatoes are ready to use. Reserve cooking water and cook until it reaches the needed temperature.

Put the ingredients in the bread pan in this order: potato cooking water, egg, mashed potatoes, butter, sugar, milk, chives, potato starch, salt, flour, and yeast.

Place the pan in the machine and close the lid. Turn it on. Choose the sweet setting and your preferred crust color. Start the cooking process. Gently unmold the baked bread and leave to cool on a wire rack.

Slice and serve.

Nutrition:

Calories: 90calories; Total Carbohydrate: 15 g   Total Fat: 2 g

Protein: 4 g Protein: 4 g

37.   Onion Potato Bread

Preparation Time: 1 hour 20 minutes

Cooking Time: 45 minutes

Servings: 2 loaves

Ingredients:

2 tablespoon quick rise yeast

4 cups bread flour

1 1/2 teaspoon seasoned salt

3 tablespoon sugar

2/3 cup baked potatoes, mashed

1 1/2 cup onions, minced

2 large eggs

3 tablespoon oil

3/4 cup hot water, with the temperature of 115 to 125 degrees F (46 to

51 degrees C)

Directions:

Put the liquid ingredients in the pan. Add the dry ingredients, except the yeast. Form a shallow well in the middle using your hand and put the yeast.

Place the pan in the machine, close the lid and turn it on. Select the express bake 80 setting and start the machine.

Once the bread is cooked, leave on a wire rack for 20 minutes or until cooled.

Nutrition:

Calories: 160calories;

Total Carbohydrate: 44 g

Total Fat: 2 g

Protein: 6 g

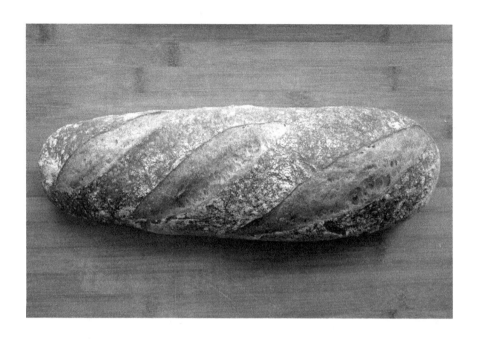

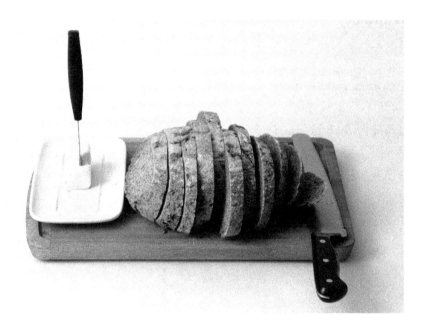

Sourdough Breads

38.   Sourdough Starter

Preparation Time: 5 days

Cooking Time:

Servings:

Ingredients:

2 cups warm water 1 tablespoon sugar 1 active dry yeast

2 cups flour 1 proper container

1 spoon for stirring

Directions:

Day 1:

Combine the water, yeast, and sugar in a medium bowl, and whisk to combine. Gently stir in the flour until well combined, and transfer to your container. Let it sit, loosely covered, in a warm spot for 24 hours.

Day 2 - 4

Unlike the traditional starter, you don't need to feed this one yet. Stir it once or twice every 24 hours.

Day 5:

By now the starter should have developed the classic slightly sour smell. If not, don't worry; you just need to let it sit a bit longer. If it is ready, store it in the fridge, and feed it once a week until you're ready to use it. As with the traditional starter, you'll need to feed it the day before you plan to use it.

Nutrition:

Calories: 26 Cal

Fat: 0 g

Carbohydrates: 6 g

Protein: 1 g

39. Garlic and Herb Flatbread Sourdough

Preparation Time: 1 hour

Cooking Time: 25- 30 minutes

Servings: 12

Ingredients:

Dough

1 cup sourdough starter, fed or unfed

3/4 cup warm water

2 teaspoons instant yeast

3 cups all-purpose flour

1 1/2 teaspoons salt

3 tablespoons olive oil

Topping

1/2 teaspoon dried thyme

1/2 teaspoon dried oregano

1/2 teaspoon dried marjoram

1 teaspoon garlic powder

1/4 teaspoon onion powder

1/4 teaspoon salt

1/4 teaspoon pepper

3 tablespoons olive oil

Directions:

Combine all the dough ingredients in the bowl of a stand mixer, and knead until smooth. Place in a lightly greased bowl and let rise for at least one hour. Punch down, then let rise again for at least one hour.

To prepare the topping, mix all ingredients except the olive oil in a small bowl.

Lightly grease a 9x13 baking pan or standard baking sheet, and pat and roll the dough into a long rectangle in the pan. Brush the olive oil over the dough, and sprinkle the herb and seasoning mixture over top. Cover and let rise for 15-20 minutes.

Preheat oven to 425F and bake for 25-30 minutes.

Nutrition:

Calories: 89 Cal

Fat: 3.7 g

Protein : 1.8 g

40. Dinner Rolls

Preparation Time: 3 hours

Cooking Time: 5-10 minutes

Servings: 24 rolls

Ingredients:

1 cup sourdough starter

1 1/2 cups warm water

1 tablespoon yeast

1 tablespoon salt 2 tablespoons sugar

2 tablespoons olive oil 5 cups all-purpose flour

2 tablespoons butter, melted

Directions:

In a large bowl, mix the sourdough starter, water, yeast, salt, sugar, and oil. Add the flour, stirring until the mixture forms a dough. If needed, add more flour. Place the dough in a greased bowl, and let it rise until doubled in size, about 2 hours.

Remove the dough from the bowl, and divide it into 2-3 inch sized pieces. Place the buns into a greased 9x13 pan, and let them rise, covered, for about an hour.

Preheat oven to 350F, and bake the rolls for 15 minutes. Remove from the oven, brush with the melted butter, and bake for an additional 5-10 minutes.

Nutrition:

Calories: 128 Cal

Fat: 2.4 g

Protein: 3.2 g

Sugar: 1.1 g

41. Sourdough Boule

Preparation Time: 4 hours

Cooking Time: 25-35 minutes

Servings: 12

Ingredients:

275g Warm Water

500g sourdough starter

550g all-purpose flour

20g Salt

Directions:

Combine the flour, warm water, and starter, and let sit, covered for at

least 30 minutes.

After letting it sit, stir in the salt, and turn the dough out onto a floured surface. It will be quite sticky, but that's okay. Flatten the dough slightly (it's best to "slap" it onto the counter), then fold it in half a few times. Cover the dough and let it rise. Repeat the slap and fold a few more times. Now cover the dough and let it rise for 2-4 hours.

When the dough at least doubles in size, gently pull it so the top of the dough is taught. Repeat several times. Let it rise for 2-4 hours once more.

Preheat to oven to 475F, and either place a baking stone or a cast iron pan in the oven to preheat. Place the risen dough on the stone or pot, and score the top in several spots. Bake for 20 minutes, then lower the heat to 425F, and bake for 25-35 minutes more. The boule will be golden brown.

Nutrition:

Calories: 243 Cal Fat: 0.7 g Protein: 6.9 g

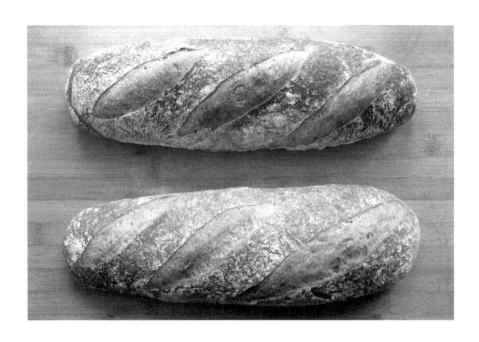

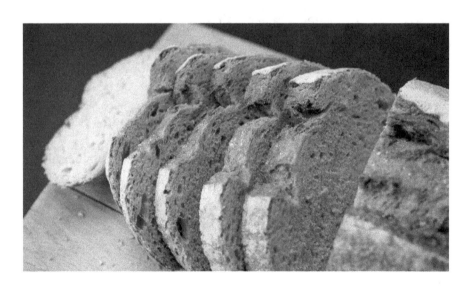

Sweet Breads

42. Brownie Bread

Preparation Time: 1 hour 15 minutes

Cooking Time: 50 minutes

Servings: 1 loaf

Ingredients:

1 egg 1 egg yolk 1 teaspoon Salt

1/2 cup boiling water

1/2 cup cocoa powder, unsweetened

1/2 cup warm water

2 1/2 teaspoon Active dry yeast

2 tablespoon Vegetable oil

2 teaspoon White sugar

2/3 cup white sugar

3 cups bread flour

Directions:

Put the cocoa powder in a small bow. Pour boiling water and dissolve the cocoa powder.

Put the warm water, yeast and the 2 teaspoon White sugar in another bowl. Dissolve yeast and sugar. Let stand for about 10 minutes, or until the mix is creamy.

Place the cocoa mix, the yeast mix, the flour, the 2/3 cup white sugar, the salt, the vegetable, and the egg in the bread pan. Select basic bread cycle. Press start.

Nutrition:

Calories: 70 Cal Fat: 3 g Carbohydrates:10 g

Protein: 1 g

43.   Black Forest Bread

Preparation Time: 2 hour 15 minutes

Cooking Time: 50 minutes

Servings: 1 loaf

Ingredients:

1 1/8 cups Warm water

1/3 cup Molasses

1 1/2 tablespoons Canola oil

1 1/2 cups Bread flour

1 cup Rye flour

1 cup Whole wheat flour

1 1/2 teaspoons Salt

3 tablespoons Cocoa powder

1 1/2 tablespoons Caraway seeds

2 teaspoons Active dry yeast

Directions:

Place all ingredients into your bread maker according to manufacture.

Select type to a light crust.

Press start.

Remembering to check while starting to knead.

If mixture is too dry add tablespoon warm water at a time.

If mixture is too wet add flour again a little at a time.

Mixture should go into a ball form, and just soft and slightly sticky to

the finger touch. This goes for all types of breads when kneading.

Nutrition:

Calories: 240 Cal

Fat: 4 g

Carbohydrates: 29 g

Protein: 22 g

44. White Chocolate Bread

Preparation Time: 3 hours

Cooking Time: 15 minutes

Servings: 12

Ingredients:

1/4 cup warm water

1 cup warm milk

1 egg

1/4 cup butter, softened

3 cups bread flour

2 tablespoons brown sugar

2 tablespoons white sugar

1 teaspoon salt

1 teaspoon ground cinnamon

1 (.25 oz.) package active dry yeast

1 cup white chocolate chips

Directions:

Put all the ingredients together, except for the white chocolate chips, into the bread machine pan following the order suggested by the manufacturer. Choose the cycle on the machine and press the Start button to run the machine. Put in the white chocolate chips at the machine's signal if the machine used has a Fruit setting on it or you may put the white chocolate chips about 5 minutes before the kneading cycle ends.

Nutrition:

Calories: 277 calories;

Total Carbohydrate: 39 g Cholesterol: 30 mg

Total Fat: 10.5 g Protein: 6.6 g

Sodium: 253 mg

Soft Breads, Vegan White

Bread, French Bread, Pumpkin

Bread ecc.

45.   Delish Soft Bread

Preparation Time: 5 minutes

Cooking Time: 3 hours

Servings: 1 loaf

Ingredients:

Water - 1 1/2 cups

1 1/2 teaspoons salt

1 tablespoon white sugar

2 1/2 teaspoons active dry yeast

Bread flour - 3 1/2 cups

Directions:

Combine the ingredients using a bread machine. Follow the order of

placement as recommended by manufacturers.

Process with basic cycle setting and light crust.

You can opt with French cycle for a crispy crust.

Let the machine do its job then serve,

Nutrition:

Calories: 60 Cal

Fat: 3 g

Carbohydrates: 10 g

Protein: 1 g

46.   Vegan White Bread

Preparation Time: 10 minutes

Cooking Time: 40 minutes

Servings: 1 loaf

Ingredients:

¼ c rice bran oil

1 c warm water

1 teaspoon salt

2 tablespoons sugar

2¼ teaspoons bread machine yeast

3 cups bread flour

Directions:

Combine sugar, yeast, and water on your bread machine pan. Set aside for about 10 minutes until it becomes frothy.

Toss in the flour, salt, and oil.

Choose the basic setting and start.

Let the machine do its job and serve.

Nutrition:

Calories: 70 Cal

Fat   : 2.2 g

Carbohydrates: 8 g

Protein : 1 g

47.   French Bread

Preparation Time: 10 minutes

Cooking Time: 40 minutes

Servings: 2 loaves

Ingredients:

1 cup Water room temperature

1 tablespoon Sugar

1 teaspoon Salt

1-1/2 teaspoon Instant Yeast

2-3/4 c Bread Flour

Directions:

Mix all ingredients in your bread machine pan.

Choose the dough cycle. Start the machine and wait until it is finished, usually for an hour and 40 mins.

After this, split the dough into 2 baguettes and cut diagonal slits across

them. Set aside, covered, for about 30 minutes.

Preheat your oven to a temperature of 190°C (375°F).

Glaze the baguette doughs with almond milk.

Pop into the oven for about 25 mins. Cool before serving.

Nutrition:

Calories: 78 Cal

Fat   : 2.9 g

Carbohydrates: 6.2 g

Protein : 1 g

48.   Spelt Bread

Preparation Time: 5 minutes

Cooking Time: 55 minutes

Servings: 1 loaf

Ingredients:

1 tablespoon oil

1 teaspoon Quick Yeast

1 teaspoon salt

1 teaspoon sugar

360ml water

500g Organic Wholemeal Spelt Flour

Directions:

Toss the ingredients in the bread machine pan.

Choose whole wheat rapid bread cycle.

Start the machine and let it do its job.

Cool the bread after the process then serve.

Nutrition:

Calories: 68 Cal

Fat   : 1.9 g

Carbohydrates: 4.2 g

Protein : 1 g

Keto Breads

49.   Best Keto Bread

Preparation Time: 10 minutes

Cooking Time: 30 minutes

Servings: 20

Ingredients:

1 ½ cup almond flour

6 drops liquid stevia

1 pinch Pink Himalayan salt

¼ tsp. cream of tartar

3 tsp. baking powder   ¼ cup butter, melted

6 large eggs, separated

Directions:

Preheat the oven to 375F.

To the egg whites, add cream of tartar and beat until soft peaks are formed.

In a food processor, combine stevia, salt, baking powder, almond flour, melted butter, 1/3 of the beaten egg whites, and egg yolks. Mix well.

Then add the remaining 2/3 of the egg whites and gently process until fully mixed. Don't over mix.

Grease a (8 x 4) loaf pan and pour the mixture in it.

Bake for 30 minutes.

Enjoy.

Nutrition:

Calories: 90 Cal

Fat: 7 g

Carbohydrates: 2 g

Protein: 3 g

50.   Yeast Bread

Preparation Time: 10 minutes

Cooking Time: 4 hours

Servings: 12

Ingredients:

2 ¼ teaspoons dry yeast

1/2 teaspoon and 1 tablespoon erythritol sweetener, divided

1 1/8 cups warm water, at 100°F / 38°C

3 tablespoons avocado oil

1 cup / 100 grams almond flour

¼ cup / 35 grams oat flour

¾ cup / 100 grams soy flour

½ cup / 65 grams ground flax meal

1 1/2 teaspoons baking powder

1 teaspoon salt

Directions:

Gather all the ingredients for the bread and plug in the bread machine having the capacity of 2 pounds of bread recipe.

Pour water into the bread bucket, stir in ½ teaspoon sugar and yeast and let it rest for 10 minutes until emulsified.

Meanwhile, take a large bowl, place the remaining ingredients in it and stir until mixed.

Pour flour mixture over yeast mixture in the bread bucket, shut the lid, select the "basic/white" cycle or "low-carb" setting and then press the up/down arrow button to adjust baking time according to your bread machine; it will take 3 to 4 hours.

Then press the crust button to select light crust if available, and press the "start/stop" button to switch on the bread machine.

When the bread machine beeps, open the lid, then take out the bread basket and lift out the bread.

Let bread cool on a wire rack for 1 hour, then cut it into twelve slices

and serve.

Nutrition:

Calories: 162 Cal

Fat: 11.3 g

Carbohydrates: 7 g

Protein : 8.1 g

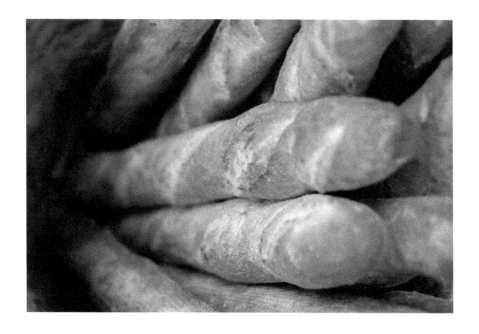

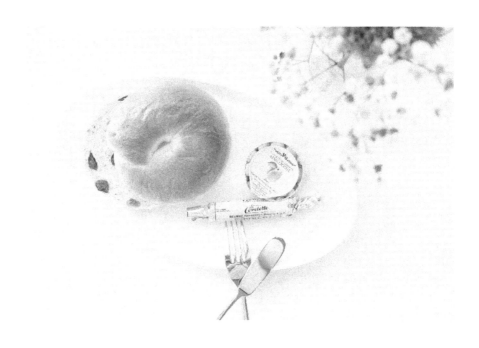

Conclusion

Depending on what kind of home baker you are, bread is either a must-know rite of passage, or an intimidating goal you haven't quite worked up the courage to try. This is because bread is a labor-intensive food where slight mistakes can have a big impact on the final result. Most of us rely on store-bought bread, but once you've tasted homemade bread, it's tempting to make your own as often as possible. A bread machine makes the process easier.

Making a loaf of bread feels like a major accomplishment. Why? There are a lot of steps. Mixing, kneading, proofing, resting, shaping, and finally baking.

You know how to make bread by hand, so how does the bread-making machine do it? A bread machine is basically a small, electric oven. It fits one large bread tin with a special axle connected to the electric motor. A metal paddle connects to the axle, and this is what kneads the dough. If you were making the bread in a mixer, you would probably use a dough hook, and in some instructions, you'll see the bread machine's kneading part referred as a hook or "blades."

The first thing you do is take out the tin and add the bread dough you made in Step 1. Bread machines can make any kind of bread, whether it's made from normal white flour, whole wheat, etc. Pop this tin unto the axle and program by selecting the type of bread, which includes options like basic, whole-wheat, multigrain, and so on. There are even cycles specifically for sweet breads; breads with nuts, seeds, and raisins; gluten-free; and bagels. Many models also let you cook jam.

You'll probably see a "dough" mode option, too. You would use that one for pizza. The machine doesn't actually cook anything; it just kneads and then you take out the pizza dough and bake it in your normal oven. If you aren't making pizza dough, the next selections you'll make are the loaf size and crust type. Once those are chosen, press the "timer" button. Based on your other selections, a time will show up and all you have to do is push "start."

After kneading and before the machine begins baking, many people will remove the dough so they can take out the kneading paddles, since they often make an indent in the finished bread. The paddles should simply pop out or you can buy a special hook that makes the removal easier. Now you can return the bread to the machine. The lid is closed during the baking process. If it's a glass lid, you can actually see what's going on. You'll hear the paddle spinning on the motor, kneading the dough. It lies still for the rising stage, and then starts again for more kneading if necessary. The motor is also off for the proving stage. Next, the heating element switches on, and steam rises from the exhaust vent as the bread bakes. The whole process usually takes a few hours.

There's a lot of work involved in making bread by hand. When you use a machine, that machine does a lot of the busy stuff for you. You just add your dough and the bread maker starts doing its thing, giving you time to do other chores or sit back and relax. As a note, not all bread makers are completely automatic, so if you want this benefit, you'll probably have to pay a bit more money. It's worth it for a lot of people, though.

Bread machines are indeed easy to use. If you can use a crockpot or a microwave, you can use a bread machine. Cycles and other settings like loaf size and color are always clearly marked, and once you do a quick read of your instruction manual, you'll be ready to go. Recipes written for bread makers are also very clear about what settings you need to select, so as long as you follow them, your bread will turn out the way you want.

CPSIA information can be obtained
at www.ICGtesting.com
Printed in the USA
BVHW040539180621
609530BV00020B/2258